# Introduction

As a practicing CRNA for eight years, I'm surprised that many of my colleagues have not considered becoming a nurse anesthetist. I did, and it was the best decision of my professional life. When I decided to pursue my certification, I wasn't sure what to expect. Like many RNs, I had heard the horror stories: "It is extremely hard," "Getting into a program is almost impossible," and "More people drop out of CRNA school than graduate." Some complain that the acceptance for a CRNA program is more stringent than a medical school. (That is an issue I will not cover as it seems to be a comparison of apples to oranges. Neither education is easy to get.)

A CRNA program is not for everyone. The path to certification is demanding, deliberately so to ensure that those who graduate are qualified to deal with the considerable responsibilities of the position. Patients who receive anesthesia expect to experience a pain-free operation and recover without complicating factors. A nurse anesthetist is "held directly responsible for maintaining their patients' physiologic parameters in the face of surgical and pharmacologic insults and not only for selecting the type of anesthetic and adjuvant drugs but also for manipulating their doses on a minute by minute basis." [i] Condensing that mouthful of words into simple terms would read, "nurse anesthetists are responsible for their patients' lives and deaths.

My purpose in authoring this book is to set the record straight, at least from one CRNA's perspective. I will cover the good, the bad, and the ugly of CRNA programs with tips to resolve some of the thornier issues that a RN considering a CRNA program might encounter.

# Chapter 1. Nursing and Anesthesia

One panoramic scene in the *Gone with the Wind* movie captured physicians and nurses as they amputated the arms and legs of screaming Civil War casualties. In the Old West, doctors required to remove bullets from a wounded hero typically resorted to long swallows of the local rotgut whiskey for patient and doctor courage. While great film scenes, such archaic techniques were relatively rare.

Few people realize that nurses have administered anesthetics - chloroform or sulfuric ether  in the United States since the Civil War. Catherine S. Lawrence is credited as the first nurse to administer an anesthetic to a Union soldier after the Battle of Bull Run.[ii]  During the latter part of the nineteenth and early twentieth centuries, anesthesia was administered primarily by nurses or medical students because physicians generally believed little training was needed.[iii]

Sister Mary Bernard Sheridan (Sisters of St. Joseph) of St. Vincent Hospital of Erie, Pennsylvania, was the first nurse to specialize in anesthesia in 1877.[iv]  In the twentieth century, government requirements for a non-physician to prescribe or administer anesthesia have been formalized and regulated in each state, as you can see in the following examples:

- **1909.** Agnes McGee established the first formal anesthesia educational program at St. Vincent's Hospital in Portland, Oregon.
- **1914.** James Gwathmey, MD issues "Anesthesia," the first authoritative book on the subject.
- **1915.** Agatha Hodgins founded the first formal postgraduate program in anesthesia at the Lakeside Hospital School of Anesthesia of Cleveland, Ohio.
- **1927.** The first medical residency for anesthesia established at the University of Wisconsin, Madison.
- **1939.** Graduates of the Lakeside School of Anesthesia established the American Association of Nurse Anesthetists (AANA).
- **1945.** First anesthesia certification exam by AANA.
- **1952.** Nurse anesthesia educational programs are accredited.
- **1956.** Certified Registered Nurse Anesthetist (CRNA) credential established.

- **1986**. Bachelor's degree in nursing or related field required to enroll in a nurse anesthesia program in the United States.
- **1990**. An entry-level CRNA required to have a master's degree in anesthesia. (In 2025, a Doctor of Nursing Practice (DNP) will be necessary.)

## What is a CRNA?

A certified registered nurse anesthetist (CRNA) is an advanced practice registered nurse who administers anesthesia and other medications to patients undergoing surgery in hospitals, clinics, and physician offices. Each CRNA has a master's degree or a higher degree specializing in anesthesiology and has completed in-depth medical training. Finally, each has passed a rigorous certification examination approved by the National Boards of Certification and Recertification of Nurse Anesthetists (NBCRNA).

CRNAs typically work with anesthesiologists, surgeons, dentists, and physicians, their relationships dictated by the laws of the state where the services are rendered.

CRNAs have specific duties, which include but are not limited to:

- Assessing patient response to anesthesia
- Identifying possible risk to the anesthetized patient, including allergies and overdose
- Administering precise dosages
- Educating patients before and after receiving anesthesia

A certified registered nurse anesthetist (CRNA) is the highest-paid advanced practice nurse, but the compensation reflects their ability to handle critical tasks, according to DailyNurse.com.[v] Wallena Gould, founder and CEO of the Diversity in Nurse Anesthesia Mentorship Program, agrees. "Our responsibility is much higher than all the other advanced practice nurses. When I tell high school students how much money we make, their eyes pop out of their heads. But the more money, the more responsibility. You literally have someone's life in your hands every day, and we make good decisions."

Of the 2.9 million registered nurses working in the United States, less than 30,000 are practicing CRNAs (about 1%). Of the nursing specialties, anesthesia administration is the most demanding and requires a multi-year journey after receiving a Bachelor of Science in Nursing (BSN) degree. Unfortunately, many capable RNs do not pursue a CRNA. Their reasons include the perception that the challenges of school, experience, and costs are too high.

Marc Code, DNP, CRNA, director of the CRNA program at Samuel Merritt University in Oakland, California, recognizes that the competition is "stiff," but not so difficult that a committed student cannot overcome the barriers.[vi] In the following pages, I will consider the obstacles you might face to become a nurse anesthetist in the United States with some tips to make your process less stressful and expensive.

## Why Become a CRNA?

I suppose, for most people, the primary reason to become a CRNA is the same reason they became an RN. Some choose nursing as a career because they want to help people, especially during periods of high stress. Others select nursing because of the pay, the opportunities in healthcare, or the base of knowledge they receive that can be applied in various situations and locations. Whatever your reason, pursuing a CRNA certification will help you achieve your goal.

CRNAs are unique because they are the primary and, often, the only providers of anesthesia care in rural America. Nurse anesthetists have always been the primary source of anesthetic care for the US military on the front lines, on ships, and in evacuation zones. According to Sonya Brown, CRNA, of western Pennsylvania, "CRNAs practice with a high degree of autonomy and carry great responsibility; consequently, they are both well-respected and well-compensated." [vii]

## Exceptional Career Satisfaction

Nurses who have achieved CRNA status report high degrees of satisfaction with their careers, possibly because they can choose the lifestyles they want. Some prefer the excitement and income opportunities in a big city trauma center. Others work in surgery centers that are open only the weekdays, so no hospital rounds and no weekends worked. My colleagues are a group of other CRNAs in Spokane, Washington, and could not dream of a more satisfying profession.

In 2019, US News & World Report ranked "nurse anesthetist" as the fifth-best profession[viii] in the country, higher than a physician (#7), veterinarian (#10), and surgeon (#17). The Medscape Nurse Career Satisfaction Report 2019[ix] found CRNAs reported that their job satisfaction was the consequence of "helping people/making a difference in peoples' lives" and "working to the full extent of my education, certification, and licensure."

## High Median Income

CRNAs are some of the highest-paid RNs in the field. Depending on the work setting and state where they are employed, the US Bureau of Labor Statistics (BLS) noted that the median annual salary for a nurse anesthetist in 2018 was $167,950, more than double the average yearly salary for an RN ($71,730).  The Table 1 below displays a range of the average salaries for CRNAs in 2020 compiled by the website Salary.com.

# Table 1 Avg CRNA Salaries 2020 from Salary.com

**How much does a Certified Nurse Anesthetist make in the United States?** The average Certified Nurse Anesthetist salary in the United States is **$186,713** as of August 27, 2020, but the range typically falls between **$171,596** and **$203,686**. Salary ranges can vary widely depending on many important factors, including education, certifications, additional skills, the number of years you have spent in your profession. With more online, real-time compensation data than any other website, Salary.com helps you determine your exact pay target.

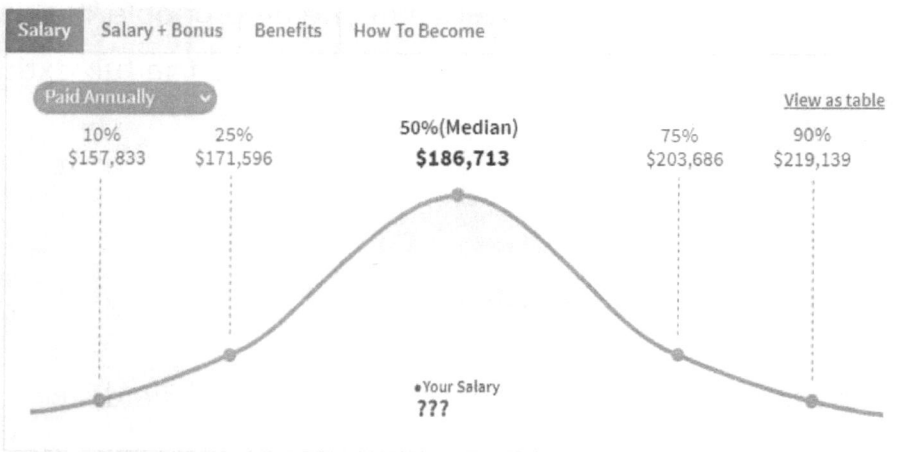

Few occupations remain unchanged by the rapid increase of technology, especially the advances in artificial intelligence (AI) and machine learning. Health care is affected by advances in diagnostic tools, new treatments, pharmaceuticals, and minimally invasive procedures resulting in less pain and quicker healing.[x] Professionals in a variety of industries have seen their jobs disappear or simplified by smart machine replacements. While the practice of a CRNA may change, the outlook for the profession remains bright. Estimates of annual growth of practicing CRNAs range from 15% to 25% (The US Department of Labor's Occupational Outlook Handbook forecasts an annual growth rate of 17%.).

An aging population and the high cost of the anesthesia care model (one anesthesiologist for every four CRNAs) today drive the demand for nurse anesthetists. [xi]

## Continuous Support System

A benefit often overlooked when deciding on a profession is your future colleagues. Operating rooms are not theater stages for divas, but the collective efforts of a well-coordinated team. When a death occurs on the OR table (and they do), colleagues who have experienced similar tragedies are needed for their sympathy and objective perspectives. To paraphrase John Donne, "No CRNA is an island entire of itself." The people you will meet are among the smartest and most caring individuals you will encounter.

## The Benefits of Diversity

Minority students will find the mentorship program started by Dr. Wallenda ("Lena") Gould especially welcoming. Diane Dy acknowledges the strength of her support system at Villanova University's CRNA program:

> *"I moved to Baltimore, MD, from the Philippines in 2006. I knew then I wanted to be a CRNA, but the task in front of me—the whole application process, going to school full time...just seems so enormous, especially when you are at a place where you do not have a lot of support. But since I attended the Diversity luncheon, to this day, that is exactly what the Diversity in Nurse Anesthesia Mentorship Program gave me—a strong support system."*

# Chapter 2. A Day in the Life of a CRNA

Nurse anesthetists work in various circumstances, including huge medical centers, community hospitals, ambulatory care centers, and physicians' offices. They work in large urban areas as well as rural towns in the least populated states of the nation. While their circumstances differ, CRNAs have similar responsibilities. During a typical day, each anesthetist performs similar duties:

## Daily Set Up of the OR

After arriving early and enjoying the first of several cups of coffee during the day, the anesthetist checks the **anesthesia machine** to ensure it is in perfect working order. (There are multiple makes and models, each requiring a unique testing process.) The check includes collecting and positioning a **suction catheter and tubing** (in case the patient vomits under sedation) and ensuring the **vital signs monitor** is functioning appropriately. The anesthetist continuously checks a patient's heart rate, oxygen saturation, respiration rate, temperature, and blood pressure during the operation.

Being prepared for the unexpected is an essential part of the job. A patient's ability to inhale and exhale through their airway must be unhindered. The CRNA pre-positions the necessary tools  a **laryngoscope handle and blade**, multiple-sized **endotracheal tubes** and **oropharyngeal airways**, a **peripheral nerve stimulator**, and **rolls of surgical ta**pe  within easy reach. If an emergency occurs, time is critical.

Finally, the setup includes a primary and backup drug set up. A typical set up includes **Midazolam** for anxiolysis and amnesia, **Fentanyl** for pain, **Lidocaine** for muscle relaxation, **Propofol** for sleepiness, and **Succinylcholine**, **Rocuronium**, or **Vecuronium** to limit movement during the operation. The secondary drugs (which you hope are not necessary) are **Phenylephrine** and **Ephedrine** in cases of low blood pressure, **Atropine** for slow heart rates, and **Esmolol** for high heart rates.

# Completing Preoperative Evaluations

The preoperative evaluation's primary purpose is to determine if the chosen procedure and anesthesia are safe and appropriate for the patient and to identify potential complications that could arise during surgery related to the patient's physical or medical condition. Before the operation (usually the evening before), the anesthetist will review the patient's **medical history**, the results of a recent **medical examination**, and meet with the patient to allay fears, discuss **anesthetic options** (general, regional, or nerve bloc), and understand the **patient's wishes** regarding optional conditions during and after the surgery).

Anesthetists typically follow a written checklist during a pre-op interview to ensure the procedures necessary to keep a patient safe are followed. Patients sometimes resent being asked questions that they have answered before and repeatedly on the day of the surgery. As hard as it might be to believe, wrong body sites, patients, and operations do occasionally occur (about one in every 112,000 procedures in the United States). When they do occur, the cause is more likely an exceptionally hectic surgery schedule that might occur after a natural disaster or similar events.

In today's litigious times, an essential consequence of the preoperative interview is securing the patient's consent for the operation to be performed on after being fully advised of the risks and possible adverse outcomes.

## Providing Anesthesia

Kelsey Horton[xii], a CRNA in Kansas, provides an apt description of the time in the OR: "I take my patient back to the operating room, induce them under anesthesia, and intubate them for the case if necessary. Throughout the procedure, I monitor the patient's vital signs, administer a variety of medications, manage the ventilator, and keep them asleep and happy. When the procedure is finished, I wake the patient up and take them to the recovery room to be cared for by the PACU nurse."

The average time for a surgical operation in America is less than an hour but varies significantly depending on the surgery, the surgeon's experience, complications, and the patient's condition. For example, there are about 500,000 percutaneous coronary intervention surgeries (PCI) each year. The surgery to open the coronary arteries to supply blood to the heart can take as little 3o minutes or several hours. Each operation requires the on-site presence of an anesthetist or anesthesiologist.

A CRNA might be in the operating room for a full day, repeating the process each time for multiple surgeries or having fewer but longer stints for more complicated operations. When outside the OR, they may be called on to place regional anesthesia blocks before and after surgeries for pain, central and arterial lines, labor epidurals and spinals, and intubations in ERs and ICUs.

## Maintaining Professional Expertise

Like all medical professionals, nurse anesthetists are required to be current with the latest medical advances and treatments that affect their practice. This requirement requires hours of reading medical and anesthetic journals, attending seminars, and regularly completing professional training programs. Each CRNA must renew their certification every eight years which requires at least 100 continuing education credits in a four-year cycle, or 25 credits each year.

# Chapter 3. The Trend to CRNA Independent Practice

In 2011, surgeon Jeffrey Parks recognized that the cost of healthcare must be controlled to prevent bankrupting our country.[xiii] Studies suggest that the cost of care per capita in the United States ($9,403) is almost double the amount spent by any other nation without corresponding indicators of better outcomes.[xiv] "Time and again, we see evidence that the amount of money we spend on health care in this country is not gaining us comparable health benefits," adds Dr. David Blumenthal, president of the Commonwealth Fund.

The cause of the excess cost is high pricing, according to many researchers. For example, primary care doctors in the United States earn, on average, $218,173, while their German and Swedish counterparts make $154,126 and $86,607, respectively. Some of the excess costs can be attributed to the artificial barriers that exist to protect certain medical specialties, including anesthesiologists (MDs who administer anesthesia). As a practicing CRNA, there is no discernable difference between what I do and the practice of a board-certified anesthesiologist. We do the exact same pre-op procedures, the same OR methods, use the same tools, keep the same charts, and, in most states, have the same DEA license.

Medical doctors attempt to justify the premium income they receive ($208,000 average in 2018) above the income of nurse anesthetists ($160,250 average in 2018) with the claim that their service provides a higher level of patient safety. Their claim is not valid. Multiple studies have shown that there is "no significant difference in the quality of care when the anesthetic is delivered by a certified registered nurse anesthetist or by an anesthesiologist." [xv] The New York Times opined on September 6, 2011, that:

"In the long run, there also could be savings to the health care system if nurses delivered more of the care. It costs more than six times as much to train an anesthesiologist as a nurse anesthetist, and anesthesiologists earn twice as much a year, on average, as the nurses do ($150,000 for nurse anesthetists and $337,000 for anesthesiologists, according to a Rand Corporation analysis)."

Dr. Parks apparently agrees with the Times, noting that, "recent studies have confirmed what everyone else in the OR already knew—that it didn't really matter who was behind the drape while a cholecystectomy was ongoing— is hardly a surprise."

For years, state legislatures have wrestled with the roles and relationship of nurse anesthetists and anesthesiologists. Three different models developed and can be found in various states today:

- **Supervision.** This model, predominant for years, means that a physician—the surgeon in the operating room (OR) or an anesthesiologist—must remain immediately available to the CRNA in case of an issue with the patient.
- **Medically directed**. Sometimes called the "team care approach," the anesthesiologist initially talks with the patient, outlines the anesthetic plan that will follow, and is present in the OR during critical moments. The Doctor then performs a post evaluation of the patient. The anesthesiologist can supervise four CRNAs simultaneously. Medicare defines seven requirements that must be met for the anesthesiologist's reimbursement.
- **CRNA Independent Practice**. Only specific states allow CRNA to work independently of a physician or anesthesiologist. In other states, the CRNA works

under the direction of a physician or dentist without an anesthesiologist's presence or control.

As time has passed with evidence of similar care and outcomes at lower costs, more states are moving to the Independent Practice model. Currently, 30 states – the most recent being Arizona in 2020 – allow CRNAs to practice skills without a physician's intervention.

# Chapter 4. CRNA Educational Preparation

You might choose to become a nurse for various reasons, including "wanting to help people" to "having a secure income." Whatever your reason, becoming a nurse can be extremely rewarding or disappointing. Nurses see patients and their families in their worse moments – scared, angry, confused – and must remain objective yet compassionate, direct, but flexible.

Nurses typically see patients more often and for more extended periods than their physicians. Understanding the unique nurse/patient relationship, Sister Marie Simone Roach, a graduate of St. Joseph's Hospital School of Nursing in 1944, defined the 5 Cs of caring as core traits of the nursing profession. You may recognize some of your own characteristics in her list:

- **Commitment**. "The life of a nurse can be challenging at times, commitment to patients cannot be sacrificed... The act of committing yourself to work means going above and beyond normally expected behaviors and pledging to uphold strong values."

22

- **Conscience**. "Conscience helps guide your actions even when focus on stress or personal matters can challenge the consistent application of best practices... Moral practices don't just arise from a strong internal sense of what's right; they also come from a continued focus on empathy and putting yourself in the patient's shoes."
- **Competence**. "Hold yourself to a high standard of excellence when fulfilling daily tasks, regardless of the behavior of others or the circumstances... Keep up-to-date with new industry developments. Learning is a lifelong activity that will serve nurses well in the ever-evolving health care field."
- **Compassion**. "Having compassion is essential for anyone in the health care profession as it takes compassion to give patients a positive experience... The more that nurses nurture their sense of compassion, the more compassion grows (and the greater positive effect it has on patient care and work relationships)."
- **Confidence**. "Confidence in experiences, education, and skills will ensure that nurses continually put their best foot forward. A confident nurse can help patients and family members deal with difficult news, and a

strong sense of self will invoke positive change in patient care."

Those who seek to practice at the highest levels of the nursing profession will consider pursuing an anesthetist certification, the CRNA. The first step on the path to certification is acceptance in one of the 121 (as of 2019) accredited nurse anesthesia programs in the United States and Puerto Rico. The programs are highly selective, but anyone with a Bachelor of Science in Nursing degree (BSN) can apply and be accepted. A list of accredited programs available in 2020 can be found on the all-crna-school website.

# CRNA Program Admission Requirements

Obtaining a CRNA is only possible through graduation from one of the accredited programs. The admission requirements are high due to the life and death responsibility that a CRMA assumes. The following preconditions are standard:

## Mandatory

- Bachelor of Science in Nursing,
- Registered Nursing License
- One-two years of critical care or ICU experience
- Cumulative GPA of 3.0 on a 4.0 system

## Typical

- Combined minimum GRE score of 300
- Prerequisite classes identified by the specific CRNA program
- Certifications determined by the CRNA program (typically a CCRN)

Graduates of the CRNA program earn either a Master of Science in Nursing (MSN) or a Doctor in Nursing Practice (DNP) depending upon their degree (BSN or MSN) when entering the program. Students entering the program after 2022 will be required to earn a doctorate (DNP) before receiving certification,

# Step 1. Gaining a BSN

I know as an RN myself that there are many excellent RNs who do not have four-year college degrees as well as high school and college graduates without a BSN who are attracted to nursing and the anesthesia programs. While their journey will be a little longer than those with a BSN, there are programs to facilitate the process.

## RNs with Associate Degrees in Nursing (ADN)

Many elect to use the ADN to become RNs because it takes about one half of the time (two years) to get a BSN (four years). Graduates of either program become RNs after passing the NCLEX exam, also known as the National Council Licensure Examination. Both programs contain the core courses and clinicals to provide graduates with hands-on learning with real patients in healthcare settings. As registered nurses, they work side-by-side, administering patient care, updating medical charts, and monitoring patients' symptoms.

The significant discernable difference is a slightly higher income - $6,000 per year according to a MedStar salary survey in 2015 – and more job opportunities for the nurses with a BSN. ADNs tend to be employed in nursing care facilities, retirement communities, outpatient clinics and assisted living facilities. BSNs are in the majority as nurses, nurse educators in colleges, and with insurance carriers as case managers.[xvi] On the other hand, the lower costs and less time required for an ADN is a financial advantage and allows its holders to join the workforce sooner.

RNs who lack a BSN degree can pursue BSN or MSN degrees to be accepted in a CRNA program. Sometimes referred to as a "bridge program," it is specially designed to consider the nursing experience and fast track the degree process. According to the All Nursing Schools website, "Bridge programs are inherently fast-paced and intense because they're geared toward students who are motivated and committed to completing their degree as quickly as possible." Those who have not practiced nursing for a while may find the course work especially challenging.

An RN to BSN can be completed in as little as twelve months because the programs typically build on the student's experience and basic nursing courses that were previously taken. The courses needed to complete the BSN degree requirements include Informatics in Nursing, Innovations in Healthcare, Nursing Management and Leadership, Nursing Ethics, Community Health, and a capstone course.

Many colleges offer online courses that can be completed at the student's own pace and exclude clinicals if the student is working as a full-time RN. In some cases, the RN's employer may reimburse tuition costs for the increased flexibility of RN assignments.

## Programs for College Non-Nursing Graduates

Many college graduates elect to become RNs after they have received degrees in other fields. Colleges have developed programs that are designed to build upon their existing degree and transition to a RN with a BSN. Often called accelerated programs, they are like bridge programs in that they consider previous education and experience. Students who pursue an accelerated program focus on nursing courses and clinical experience. They typically have completed the Arts and Social Science requirements, but lack the Natural Science courses like Anatomy, Microbiology, and Chemistry.

Students in accelerated programs should be prepared for full-time, onsite attendance with 90 laboratory hours and 660 hours of clinical training on direct patient care.

Completion of the program typically requires twelve to eighteen months.

## College Students Pursuing a BSN

Career counselors generally recommend that students interested in nursing attend a university or college with a Bachelor of Science in Nursing program and subsequently become RNs. Over 80% of new nurses entering the profession today hold a BSN, and there were more nurses with BSNs than ADNs for the first time in 2015.
Many regulatory bodies and nursing associations advocate that anyone seeking to be an RN has a BSN. If you anticipate applying for a CRNA program later, you will need a four-year Bachelor of Science in Nursing degree.

The website RNcareers identified more than 930 BSN degree programs in the United States. A sample of the number of CRNA programs, average NCLEX passing rate, and cost of attendance is available in the Appendix. Prospective students need to ensure that their chosen school is accredited by the Accreditation Commission for Education in Nursing (ACEN) or the Commission on Collegiate Nursing Education (CCNE). Accreditation is essential due to its effects on the student's

- Ability to transfer credits to other schools
- Access to financial aid and grants
- Ability to take licensing exams
- Access to jobs

Schools may have a national accreditation, regional accreditation, or both. A student transferring between a nationally accredited school and a regionally accredited school, and vice versa, may have problems transferring credits. This is particularly the case if they are moving from one region to another.

Accreditation is not automatic. A school may lose accreditation if it fails to maintain the quality and requirements of the accreditation authority.

## Step 2. Maximize Your BSN Experience

A Bachelor of Science in Nursing degree is typically earned over four curriculum years (Freshman, Sophomore, Junior, Senior). Students take a combination of science (Chemistry, Anatomy, Nutrition, Microbiology), liberal arts (English, Sociology, Anthropology), and specialized nursing courses. Like other STEM degrees, the courses required for graduation are demanding. Some students suggest that two to four hours of study is necessary for each hour of lecture or lab.

Many people do not realize the various types of nursing degrees available or the requirements to receive certification (Table 2. details educational requirements, average income, and typical duties for each type).

## Table 2 Types of Nursing Degrees

| Nursing Degrees* | | | |
|---|---|---|---|
| Type | Nursing Assistant CNA | Licensed Practical Nurse (LPN) | Registered Nurse (RN) | Advanced Practice Registered Nurse (APRN) |
| Education | State-approved education program/state exam | Practical Nursing Diploma/NCLEX-PN Exam | Associate Degree in Nursing (ADN) or Bachelor of Science in Nursing (BSN)/NCLEX exam | Master's of Science in Nursing. nurse anesthetists, nurse midwives, certifieed nurse practicioners, clinical nurse specialists |
| Education Source | Nursing homes, Technical colleges, American Red Cross | Techncical, community, or career colleges | College or University | Universities Graduate Programs/State test for specilaty |
| Duties | Help pateients with physical needs, measure vital signs, dispense medicines in some states | Monitorr patient health and administer basic care (insert catheters, start IV drips, change bandages) | Direct patient care, promote public health, run health screenings, or staff clinics | All of the duties of an RN as and more extensive tasks like ordering and evaluating test results, referring patients to specialists and diagnosing and treating ailments |
| Med. Salary (2017) | $27,510 | $45,030 | $70,000 | $110,930 |
| Ann. Growth | 11% | 12% | 15% | 31% |

*Malvik, C, A Beginner's Guide to Understanding the Levels of Nursing Credentials. Rasmussen College, January 7, 2019.

Just getting by is not good enough if you are aiming to become a nurse anesthetist. Good grades are essential for those who pursue a CRNA after their BSN. A 3.0 GPA ("B") is the minimum generally accepted by a CRNA graduate program, though some schools may consider any exceptional circumstances that might apply to you.

Take full advantage of your college years to make an impressive resume (honor societies, academic awards, dean's list, professional organizations). Take optional courses that will add critical care experience, At a minimum, join the National Student Nurses Association and be as active as possible without jeopardizing your studies.

Some CRNA schools may ask you for personal references. It is always a good idea to make and maintain contacts with the professional people who help you during your college and early professional years. There is no hard and fast rule about references regarding their professional position or standing. Some programs might ask for a referral from an instructor or dean from your college; others prefer someone who has more recent experience with you. Others might ask for recommendations from a physician or a practicing CRNA. The critical criteria for the choice of the person writing a recommendation are that they

1. agree to write and deliver the reference promptly,
2. practice acceptable writing skills, and
3. know you well enough to describe your skills and accomplishments.

If you ask someone for a reference, be sure and follow up with a personal, hand-written, "thank you" note. Busy people – the ones you want as references – take the time to complete a referral. Show your appreciation.

## Step 3. Pass the NCLEX-RN Exam

The NCLEX exam, also known as the National Council Licensure Examination, is a standardized test that every state regulatory board uses to determine if a candidate is ready to become licensed as an entry-level nurse. Nursing students must complete their respective nursing programs before they can sit for an NCLEX examination. After the nursing authority of the testing state declares the candidate eligible for testing, they receive an Authorization to Test that identifies the candidate's authorization number, identification number, and expiration date by which the test must be taken.

Most questions on the exam are multiple-choice, but other formats such as "fill in the blank" have been added in recent years. The minimum/maximum number of questions on the test for RNs is 85/265, with a six-hour maximum time limit to complete.[xvii] Test examinees do not receive a number grade, but a "Pass" or "Fail." First-time pass rates for those with a BSN are historically between 86%-90%.

Each state has its own specific requirements to sit for the examination, so potential applicants should contact their state Board of Nursing to determine the latest requirements. In some cases (Delaware and Virginia), nurses applying from out-of-state schools must have 440-500 clinical hours before they can sit for an examination. Some states require proof of US citizenship and criminal background checks.

While not mandatory, many schools urge students who will take the NCLEX to utilize the Practice Exams developed by the National Council of State Boards of Nursing, Inc. (NCSBN). Most recommend a study guide, such as the Saunders Comprehensive Review for the NCLEX-RN Examination.

Following the successful completion of the NCLEX, you are ready to accept your first full-time position as a registered nurse.

# Step 4. Pass the Graduate Record Exam (GRE)

Nurses with a BSN and expectation to pursue a specialized certification or higher professional degrees (MSN or DNP) might be required to take and pass the GRE before acceptance into a CRNA program or graduate school. Some schools require the GRE only for nurse practitioners who do not meet the minimum GPA. Others recommend that students with satisfactory GRE scores submit them to be considered holistically with other admissions qualifications.

## When to Take the Test

You should consider taking the GRE as soon as possible after passing the NCLEX, even if you will not apply to a CRNA program for several years. The score you receive is valid for five years from the day you take the test, although some schools might require a GRE score earned within two  three years of admission.

My experience is that the longer you are away from school and regular testing, your proficiency in test-taking declines. Today's competency in GRE skills is not going to be at the same level you had five years earlier. If you take the GRE and then spend the next five years without even looking at a number, you should expect to brush up to get back your quantitative skills. (Some research claims that if you are not using the skills at all, you will lose your edge much more quickly than five years.) However, it is also possible that your work experience and increased knowledge will improve your score, so your decision is not clear-cut unless you plan to pursue a Master of Science in Nursing shortly after your BSN graduation.

## GRE General Test

Most applicants to a graduate school are required to take the GRE General Test administered by the Educational Testing Service (ETS). The test consists of three sections: verbal reasoning, quantitative reasoning, and analytical writing with four types of questions – multiple choice with one answer, multiple choice with plural answers, calculations, and comparisons. The analytical writing section requires essay answers.

Most students complete the test within three-and-a-half to four hours. Though the three sections of the test are individually scored, graduate schools may consider the applicant's score and percentile ranking (how your performance compares to the other test-takers) in each section. According to ETS, the mean score of all GRE test-takers (2015-2018) was 306.86. Table 3 provides an indication of the scores for each percentile of test takers.

*Table 3 GRE Scores & Percentiles - Educational Testing Service*

**GRE General Test Interpretive Data**

Percent of test takers scoring lower than selected scaled scores.

| Scaled Score | Verbal Reasoning | Quantitative Reasoning | Score Levels | Analytical Writing |
|---|---|---|---|---|
| 170 | 99% | 95% | 6.0 | 99% |
| 165 | 96% | 86% | 5.0 | 92% |
| 160 | 86% | 73% | 4.5 | 81% |
| 155 | 68% | 56% | 4.0 | 57% |
| 150 | 46% | 37% | 3.5 | 39% |
| 145 | 26% | 19% | 3.0 | 15% |

Fortunately, candidates can repeat the computerized GRE General Test up to five times each year with no limits on the paper tests. Each test costs $205, and takers can choose to report the score from a specific test date, the most recent test, or all test scores you have taken over the previous five years.

## GRE Test Preparation

Most experts suggest that you take six to eight weeks to prepare for the GRE, especially if you have been out of school for a couple of years and have a career or family. You will need to sharpen your memory as well as your test-taking skills. One of my biggest concerns was about the math skills required. To my eternal relief, I discovered the math requirements could be handled with basic algebra and statistics. Don't worry about digging out old calculus books and the like,

All GRE test takers should at least take the practice tests available from ETS. Completing the tests before the real thing will familiarize you with the type of questions you can expect, the on-screen calculator that you will be using for the quantitative parts, and let you develop a time schedule that is best for you.

Everyone tests at a different speed and has different skills. Do not select a preparation strategy because it worked for someone else as you are unique. Create a plan that is best for you, and do not look back. Successful test takers are like public speakers, their best performances result from a combination of self-confidence and fear. You will need to find your own "sweet spot" to excel at the task before you.

There are a variety of companies that provide test preparation for a fee. Some of the more popular suppliers include Magoosh, Kaplan, and Princeton Review. Before selecting the company to help you, ask fellow students and your instructors what GRE prep courses they recommend and consider their costs. Remember, the deciding factor in your score is your effort to prepare, not the prep course you choose.

## GRE Subject Tests

Applicants can also take subject tests to verify their mastery of a specific discipline. Nursing graduates are not required to take the tests as part of their application to graduate school but may choose to do so to differentiate their skills from other applicants. The subject tests most likely to benefit CRNA applicants are Biology and Chemistry.

# Chapter 5. MSN Before CRNA Program

While an MSN is a necessary requirement to become a CRNA, the degree can be earned before entering CRNA school or the result of completing a CRNA program. Many BSNs enter graduate school immediately after graduation rather than wait until their clinical work is over. Others prefer to work several years gaining experience and preparing financially to become a full-time student the second time. There are advantages and disadvantages to each approach and, as such, your decision is best made on your personal circumstances

## Master of Science in Nursing

A Master of Science in Nursing (MSN) is a graduate degree sandwiched between the BSN and a DNP in Nursing. Typically requiring a two- to three-year commitment, a master's degree in nursing is the first step in the credentialing process required for an anesthesia specialty. An MSN is also a requirement for a doctorate in nursing.

All MSN programs require that you have a bachelor's degree, but they do not all require that you be an RN before entering the program. A master in a nursing program is either a Master of Science in Nursing (MSN) degree or a Master of Science with a nursing major (MS). Both degree types are respected equally within the nursing profession.

According to Kathleen Poindexter, DNP, RN, CNE, ANEF, president-elect of the National League for Nursing (NLN), MSN programs offer a generalist degree or one of several specializations in a wide range of clinical and non-clinical areas. "A Master's level program is going to prepare any of these nurses with advanced specialized knowledge and skills to navigate in an area of nursing expertise." [xviii]

## MSN Admission Requirements

You should expect that graduate nursing classes will be more difficult and demanding than your undergraduate nursing classes. Having completed advanced science and anatomy is a common requirement. Applicants are generally required to have

- A BSN from an accredited program
- A current RN license

- Minimum GPA and GRE scores of 3.0 on a 4.0 scale
- Clinical experience (varies by program, usually a one-year minimum)
- Letters of academic or professional reference
- A successful personal interview

The length of time required to complete an MSN program varies according to a student's previous education, experience, specialty, and student status (part- or full-time). A full-time student pursuing a generalist MSN may complete the course in as little as eighteen months while part-time or those seeking a specialty might take three to five years.

## Joint Master's Degree Options

Some universities offer the option to combine an MSN with another graduate degree (the applicant must qualify for admission to each program). Popular combinations are

- **MSN/MPH**. A combination of a Master of Science in Nursing and a Master of Public Health (MPH) for those seeking advanced nursing skills and work within the areas of local or global public health.

- **MSN/MBA**. Combining the skills of an MSN with a Master of Business Administration prepares graduates for the business side of healthcare, whether directing their own practice or a health organization.
- **MSN/MHA**. Nurses who seek management positions in healthcare organizations can pursue an MSN and a Master of Healthcare Administration.

# Doctor of Nursing Practice Requirements for CRNAs

Students entering a CRNA Program after 2022 will be required to earn a Doctor of Nursing Practice for certification. Students with an MSN will earn a DNP as part of the CRNA program. Students with a BSN will be an accelerated DNP in their CRNA program, the difference being one to two additional years in the program.

 A DNP is not the same as a Ph.D. in Nursing. A Doctor of Nursing Practice focuses on the clinical side of healthcare, while a Ph.D. deals more with research and education.

## DNP versus MD

While both credentials represent a significant accomplishment and take years to achieve, the two are vastly different in training, scope, and responsibilities. Their training is different, as are their specialties. Ironically, when a CRNA administers anesthesia to a patient, it is considered a "nursing practice;" if an MD anesthesiologist administers anesthesia, it is a "medical practice" even though the procedures and responsibilities are the same.

- **DNP**. A CRNA with a DNP degree typically spends three to five years after getting their bachelor's degree. A CRNA program usually requires a GPA between 3.0-3.2. Only some schools require a GRE score, and its weight in the evaluation of applicants is less than the influence of an MCAT score for prospective physicians.
- **MD**. A physician spends an additional nine to eleven years after getting their bachelor's degrees. The typical medical school requires an undergraduate GPA of 3.60 or higher and an MCAT (the equivalent of the GRE for medical school) score in the top ten percentile. An MD specializing in anesthesia – an

anesthesiologist – earns about twice as much as a nurse anesthetist.

## Use of the "Doctor" Title

The honorific "Doctor" can be used by anyone who has earned the academic or professional designation. Physicians, dentists, and veterinarians are regularly addressed as Doctor. Those who have earned PhDs in other professions are often called Doctors, such as college professors, religious teachers, and pharmacists. Anyone who has earned a DNP is entitled to use the title.

Whether or not the title should be used by DNPs in a medical setting remains controversial. In such contexts, most people (and patients) are likely to assume the title refers to a physician and that the holder has an MD. For this reason, many DNPs do not use the title. Miriam Yazai of nurse.org provides insight into the issue and concludes, "No matter who you are or where you stand on each argument, it can be said that ego lies at the center of the feud." Like Yazai, I will leave what you prefer to be called and under what circumstances to you.

# Chapter 6. CRNA Clinical Requirements

The Council on Accreditation Nurse Anesthesia Educational Programs mandates that CRNA programs require incoming students to have at minimum one year of critical care nursing experience. The schools prefer students with work experience that will aid them in the field of anesthesia  a knowledge that can only be gained by working in the ICU setting

Most CRNA programs seek candidates who have managed gravely ill patients on ventilators with invasive monitoring, vasopressor infusions, and other resuscitative efforts. It is crucial to ensure your experience working as a nurse is preparing you for success in nurse anesthesia school.

## Acceptable Critical Care Experience

It is best to get this experience in an ICU unit in a hospital or a surgical intensive care unit (SICU). The latter is preferred since SICU nurses work with patients who had a coronary artery bypass graft (CABG). SICU experience gives you in-depth knowledge of physiology, anatomy, pharmacology, and assessment skills.

Generally, acceptable critical care experience typically includes ICU (Intensive Care Unit), SICU (Surgical Intensive Care), MICU (Medical Intensive Care), CVICU (Cardiovascular Intensive Care), PICU (Pediatric Intensive Care Unit), CCU (Coronary Care Unit), or CTICU (Cardio-Thoracic Intensive Care Unit). Each program determines its own criteria for admission.

Experiences that are typically NOT accepted by CRNA programs include OR (Operating Room), PACU (Post Anesthesia Care Unit), NICU (Neonatal Intensive Care), Cardiac Step-down, Telemetry, or Emergency Room (ER).

## Tips to Find CCU Positions

Many hospitals require experience in a critical care environment before employment in a critical care unit, creating a dilemma for new RNs. Finding a position in critical care shortly after receiving your RN can be difficult. But, with creativity, persistence, and flexibility, new RNs can obtain critical care positions:

- **Internships**. Some hospitals offer internships, provide training, and hire promising participants for critical care positions.
- **Tech/CNA positions**. Some nurses claim the best way to get a job in an ICU is as a tech/CNA. Remember, hospitals look at internal candidates before looking at external candidates. The nurse manager will be familiar with your work, so hiring you as an RN will be viewed with less risk.
- **Teaching hospitals**. Many offer programs for RNs new to critical care.
- **Overlooked hospitals**. Small, rural, and inner-city hospitals are typically less competitive than their larger urban counterparts.

## Certifications

In addition to gaining valuable critical care nursing experience, most CRNA schools want their applicants to have some specific certifications, which verify your knowledge and competence in the respective areas. The following certifications may not all be required by every nurse anesthesia program, but many are.

While some of the following certifications are not a requirement for a CRNA program, an employer typically expects the certifications to be completed within three to six months after hiring. Since many hospitals will reimburse the cost of required certifications (BLS, PALS, ACLS), some career counselors recommend waiting until employment to get the certifications. Otherwise, the applicant will bear the costs.

- **BLS (Basic Life Support).** Hospitals require this certification for all RNs. The certification is through the American Heart Association. The course focuses on life-saving care such as CPR, the use of an automated external defibrillator (AED), and removal of airway obstructions.
- **ACLS (Advanced Cardiac Life Support).** The certification is required for RNs who work in the ER or ICU. The course covers the management of respiratory and cardiac arrest, airway management, intubation, communications, and membership on a resuscitation team.
- **PALS (Pediatric Advanced Life Support).** The certification confirms the holder as competent to provide life-giving care to infants and children

(excluding critically ill neonates and within an NICU setting).

# Critical Care Registered Nurse (CCRN)

Having a CCRN certification might help the chances of being admitted into a CRNA program. According to Dr. Charnelle Lewis, DNP, CRNA, having a CCRN is becoming the standard for many schools.

This certification is not a requirement to work in a critical care setting, but it is evidence that the holder can function effectively under stress. The certification is "the initial building block towards becoming a certified registered nurse anesthetist (CRNA)." Ari Newman, a RN for thirteen years, recalls that the three-hour, 150-question test is difficult and recommends a combination of review courses and live workshops for preparation.

An RN seeking CRNA certification must have a

- minimum of 1,750 hours of direct bedside care in a critical care area in the immediate prior two-year period with 875 hours in the most recent month, or

- practice for a minimum of five years, 2000 hours in direct bedside care of critically ill patients (144 hours in the most recent twelve months).[xix]

# Other Certifications That Make a Difference

Other certifications that look good to schools include the TNCC (Trauma Nursing Core Course), CMC (Cardiac Medicine Certification), and CSC (Cardiac Surgery Certification). Both the CMC and CSC are additions to your CCRN. Once you have acquired your CCRN, you are eligible to take the test. Since few applicants will have the certification, it will make your application stand out.

# Important RN Organizations

Once you are a practicing RN, join the American Nurses Association for networking opportunities and a chance to get your opinions heard. Two other organizations that warrant membership are the American Association of Critical Care Nurses (AACN) and the Emergency Nurses Association (ENA). Working in an emergency room is not required for membership.

# Chapter 7. CRNA Admission

Joining a CRNA program is like becoming a member of other elite groups known for their professionalism, accomplishments, and reputations. Acceptance is difficult because it is reserved for the best in the profession  the rare few who are willing to perform the necessary work to achieve proficiency,

"This is probably one of the most rewarding fields in nursing, and almost [every CRNA] has a high level of job satisfaction. But that also makes it the most competitive," says Henry Talley V, Ph.D., CRNA, MSN, MS, BA, director of the newly accredited CRNA program at Michigan State University College of Nursing. "Meeting the minimum standards does not give you a good chance of getting into a program [that can only accept] 10 or 15 students. You really want to have at least a 3.5 GPA, with excellent grades in your science courses and in your last two years. If your GPA is lower, you need to do very well on your GRE." [xx]

# Program Selection

Demand for nurse anesthetists is high enough that many CRNAs claim the choice of programs will not affect the job opportunities or compensation of any graduate. Nevertheless, the decision of the place that you will live and work for three to five years is important. In addition to such factors as costs, location, and financial aid, you should consider

- **Passing and placement rates.** The more popular schools invariably have higher rates than others due to their visibility in the hospital community, the number and success of alumni, and the professional stature of teachers and instructors. These advantages do not preclude smaller, less-known programs from providing an excellent education and experience. Remember that everyone must pass the same certification exams.
- **Faculty credentials.** Professional reputation is not an indication of excellent instruction. Do not be awed by credentials unless they specifically relate to teaching. My best teachers were those who took the time to be sure I understood the lesson.

- **Student to Teacher ratio**. The typical student/teacher ratio for CRNA programs is thirteen to eighteen students to one teacher. If instructors deal with fewer students, they theoretically have more time to spend per student. Schools with higher ratios may expect students to progress more independently.
- **Learning style**. Some program mix classroom and clinicals instruction, such as three months in a classroom followed by a period of clinicals and repeat. Others complete the academic coursework before beginning clinicals. If you have a preference, you need to consider the system used in the individual CRNA programs.

If possible, try to visit your top two or three CRNA program candidates before choosing a favorite. Nothing beats face-to-face conversations with students and faculty in their environment to get a feel of how you might fit.

Some people complain that being accepted in a CRNA program is more selective than med school. "We're very selective, but we lose very few students—usually only one or two each year," says Sass Elisha, CRNA, EdD, academic and clinical educator at Kaiser Permanente School of Anesthesia in Pasadena, California confirms that CRNA programs are very selective and notes, "The people that apply are unbelievably high-quality students. Their knowledge base and scholarship are impressive, and that makes it very difficult to analyze applicants."

## Relocation as a Possibility

Living and practicing on the West Coast, I am frequently asked, "What is the best way to get into a school?" The secret is to move to areas with more programs. Pennsylvania has a dozen schools with CRNA programs, and Texas has five schools. There are more schools in the East than on the West Coast. Acceptance may require moving to find an opening. I found the Council on Accreditation's website – CRNA School Search – invaluable in my search for information about programs.

## Multiple Applications

There are no limits to the number of CRNA programs where a student might apply other than a financial and logical limit. Each school requires a non-refundable application fee that ranges from $50 to $125. Applicants should also consider the likelihood of being accepted based on their credentials (popular programs are typically highly selective).

Most experts recommend filing three to five applications at most.

## Financial Assistance

There are government loans available for college students, including those in CRNA programs. However, student loans under current law must be repaid under all circumstances, even after personal bankruptcy. Students should carefully consider the advantages and disadvantages of assuming student debt. Various scholarships and grants are available from organizations like the American Association of Nurse Anesthetists, the Anesthesia Patient Safety Foundation, and multiple state organizations.

The US Military will pay for your CRNA training in return for active service after graduation. The US Army, for instance, offers a Graduate Program in Anesthesia Nursing for nurses serving in the Army Nurse Corps. The Army pays tuition and educational expenses, and students also receive full Army pay. Military CRNAs serve in combat zones and must meet military standards unrelated to their nursing duties.

# CRNA Personal Essay

Your essay is your best opportunity to show off your experiences and detail why you would be an exceptional addition to the CRNA program. It is your chance to sell yourself, and you do not want to blow it with an unintended error. Here are some tips to make your essay stand out:

1. **Stay within required word limits**. An unwillingness or inability to follow simple directions is a killer. It is also a test of your analytical skills, knowing what is essential and what is trivial. Have several people – preferably nurses or academics - read your drafts to ensure conciseness and cohesion.

2. **Avoid grammatical and spelling errors**. Nothing turns off readers like misuse of tenses, bad punctuation, or misspelled words. Use simple sentences and avoid polysyllabic words when possible to facilitate understanding, i.e., do not take fifteen words to say what you could in eight words. Use proofreaders to catch errors as well as a program like Grammarly.

3. **Explain your reasons for becoming a CRNA.** If possible, relate your motive to something or someone

in your life that sparked your desire. Wanting to make more money or practice autonomously are not good reasons! Give the admissions committee cause to like you and help you achieve your goal. This section is also your opportunity to explain why you chose to apply to the specific CRNA program. Compliments are always appreciated unless they are blatantly false.

4. **Detail your critical care experience**. Your essay should include your typical patients' acuity, experience with ventilators, vasoactive drips, Swanz Ganz, etc., and your participation in any emergency acute care teams.

5. **Include lessons learned**. Identifying a significant failure and what you learned can be powerful and a demonstration that you are willing to learn. One caution: do not include more than one or two examples, or you risk the appearance of being regularly unprepared to fulfill your responsibilities.

If you have writer's block or do not know where to start, search the Internet with the term "CRNA Admission Essay" to find good and bad examples of previous CRNA applicants. Your search may trigger ideas for your essay.

# Applicant Interview

The program interview is usually your first (and possibly your only) opportunity to sell yourself to the admissions committee. Being prepared is essential if you want to make a winning impression. The conclusions that individual committee members make are subjective, and the judging begins when you walk through the door. I have sat on many selection committee interviews, leading to my recommendations to an applicant going through the process:

1. **First impressions matter.** Humans are predisposed to make quick judgments, often with little information. A survey by HR Daily Advisor found that almost one-half of employers decide whether a candidate is a good or bad fit within five minutes of meeting; less than 10% took as long as 30 minutes to reach a conclusion. Another study found that attractiveness, likeability, competence, trustworthiness, and aggressiveness are evaluated in the first few seconds or less. Do not ruin your chances by a messy appearance, wearing inappropriate clothes, or acting in a cavalier manner.

2. **Be prepared**. While some programs treat the interview as a "meet and greet" event without difficult questions, my experience (and I expect the same for most CRNA programs) is that the meeting is intense and probing. We ask tough clinical questions that range from human and disease processes, pharmacology, and anatomy to the interpretation of lab results. A candidate should be able to answer these clinical questions without difficulty if they adequately prepared for the interview.

3. **Curb your ego**. The other portion of the interview process is subjective and designed to see if applicants will be able to work effectively as team members. Most CRNA applicants have Type A personalities. They have been a nurse for several years and are at the apex of their nursing communities. Many have massive egos and may be confrontational with the professors and personnel at the clinical sites. Our concerns are such that some programs have a psychologist sit in on the interview to evaluate a student's nonverbal communication.

Learn and remember your interviewers' names and follow the interview with a hand-written, personal "thank you" to each of the interviewers. A personal touch shows respect and brings your name to the forefront one more time.

# Chapter 8. Final Thoughts

Getting accepted into a CRNA program is just the beginning of your journey. More than any other nursing education program, earning an MSN or Doctor of Nursing degree in anesthesia requires you to totally commit to your studies. The pace is fast, the classes are rigorous, and the clinical portion is so time-intensive that it feels like a full-time job. You will be living, eating, and breathing CRNA for 24 to 36 months, depending on your program's length.

With few exceptions, all accredited CRNA programs are full time. Students are usually prohibited, or at least discouraged, from working. During the clinical phase of the program, you will not have time to work, even part-time. A student who is also a parent should arrange fail-safe childcare to avoid interruptions during critical clinical tours.

"Many nurses don't recognize the true rigors of the program and are unprepared when clinicals start," says Gould, the LaSalle University Nurse Anesthesia Program graduate. "You need to realize that you'll be taking at least two exams a week. You'll be challenged verbally all day during clinicals. Instructors will be asking you, 'What are you going to do?

Why are you doing it? How would you do it differently if the patient had asthma?'"

Admission standards and study requirements are high because of the life and death responsibility of a CRNA. The period of training is one of the most grueling experiences a nurse will have. There is no substitute for being prepared beforehand. One CRNA graduate remembered, "After a time, I realized that you can get through it either by casting yourself into it whole-heartedly (devoting yourself to it) or could do just enough to get by, or could even be dragged through kicking and screaming. You got through in each case but devoting yourself to it was a lot more pleasant. Win, lose or draw, I slept better at night – knowing there was nothing more I could have done to keep my patients safe... It *can* be the worst two years of your life, or you can make it the *best* two years [of your life]." [xxi]

Good luck with your applications and your studies. I look forward to welcoming you into our select community of nurse anesthetists.

# End Notes

[i] Booth MJ. Nurse anesthetist reaction to the unexpected or untimely death of patients in the operating room. *Holist Nurs Pract*. 1998;13(1):51-58. doi:10.1097/00004650-199810000-00008

[ii] Lawrence, C S. *Sketch of life and labors of Miss Catherine S. Lawrence*, (James B.Lyon Publisher, 1896), 114.

[iii] Ahmad M, Tariq R (2017) History and evolution of anesthesia education in United States. *J Anesth Clin Res*. 2017; 8: 734.

[iv] Bruce, D. Erie boasts 140 years of nurse anesthetists, Goerie website. January 14, 2017. (Accessed May18, 2020). https://www.goerie.com/news/20170114/erie-boasts-140-years-of-nurse-anesthetists

[v] Farmer, R. Why you should consider becoming a nurse anesthetist, DailyNurse website. June 14, 2016. (Accessed May 19, 2020). https://dailynurse.com/consider-becoming-nurse-anesthetist/

[vi] Farmer, R. Why you should consider becoming a nurse anesthetist, DailyNurse website. June 14, 2016. (Accessed May 19, 2020). https://dailynurse.com/consider-becoming-nurse-anesthetist/

[vii] Brown, S.  A day in the life of a CRNA. Barton Associates Blog website.  January 23, 2020 (Accessed May 19, 2020). https://www.bartonassociates.com/blog/a-day-in-the-life-of-a-crna

[viii] *US News*.  US News announces the 2019 best j,obs, *U.S. News & World report*, January 8, 2019. (Accessed May 20, 2020). https://www.usnews.com/info/blogs/press-room/articles/2019-01-08/us-news-announces-the-2019-best-jobs

[ix] Stokowski, L, McBride, M, Berry, E. *Medscape nurse satisfaction report 2019*, Medscape website. December4, 2019. (Accessed May 20, 2020). https://www.medscape.com/slideshow/2019-nurse-career-satisfaction-6012376

[x] Jones, Mi. HealthCare: How technology impacts the healthcare Industry. Medium website. December 26, 2018. https://healthcareinamerica.us/healthcare-how-technology-impacts-the-healthcare-industry-b2ba6271c4b4

[xi] MacKinnon, M. How 3 key healthcare trends affect CRNA & predictions for the future. Becker's ASC Review website. September 19, 2016. https://www.beckersasc.com/anesthesia/how-3-key-healthcare-trends-affect-crnas-predictions-for-the-future.html

[xii] Inside Look: The day-to-day of a nurse anesthetist. ATI Nursing Education website. October 12, 2017 (Accessed May 27, 2020). https://atinursingblog.com/inside-look-the-day-to-day-of-a-nurse-anesthetist/

[xiii] Parks, J. How MD anesthesiologists have become victims of their own excellence, KevinMD website. January 22,2011. https://www.kevinmd.com/blog/2011/01/md-anesthesiologists-victims-excellence.html

[xiv] Mangan, D. US healthcare spending is high. Results are...not so good, CNBC website. October 8, 2015. (Accessed May 27. 2020). https://www.cnbc.com/2015/10/08/us-health-care-spending-is-high-results-arenot-so-good.html

[xv] Editorial: Who should provide anesthesia care? *New York Times* website. (September 6, 2010). https://www.nytimes.com/2010/09/07/opinion/07tue3.html

[xvi] Bureau of Labor Statistics, US Department of Labor. *Occupational outlook handbook*. Accessed January 2, 2019 www.bls.gov/ooh/. Information represents national, averaged data for the occupations listed and includes workers at all levels of education and experience. Employment conditions in your area may vary.

[xvii] NCLEX: What is NCLEX & NCLEX requirements. RegisteredNurseRN website. (Accessed May 21, 2020). https://www.registerednursern.com/nclex-what-is-nclex-nclex-requirements/

[xviii] Earning a Master's of Nursing degree. All Nursing Schools website. (Accessed May 22, 2020). https://www.allnursingschools.com/msn/

[xix] CCRN certification. CCRNReview website. (Accessed May 22, 2020). https://www.ccrnreview.com/ccrn-certification

[xx] The minority student's guide to CRNA programs. *Minority Nurse Magazine*. March 30, 2013.

https://minoritynurse.com/the-minority-students-guide-to-crna-programs/

[xxi] Dosch, M. Quotes. University of Detroit Mercy Graduate Program in Nurse Anesthesiology website, August 2019. (Accessed May 20, 2020). https://healthprofessions.udmercy.edu/academics/na/agm/quotes.htm